Medication Tracker

Medication Name	Dosage	Frequency	Started Date	Finished Date

AF797468

Medication Tracker

Medication Name	Dosage	Frequency	Started Date	Finished Date

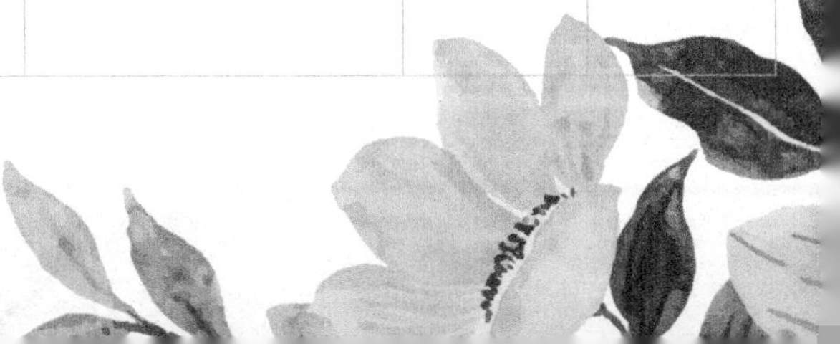

Medication Tracker

Medication Name	Dosage	Frequency	Started Date	Finished Date

Medication Tracker

Medication Name	Dosage	Frequency	Started Date	Finished Date

Medication Tracker

Medication Name	Dosage	Frequency	Started Date	Finished Date

Medication Tracker

Medication Name	Dosage	Frequency	Started Date	Finished Date

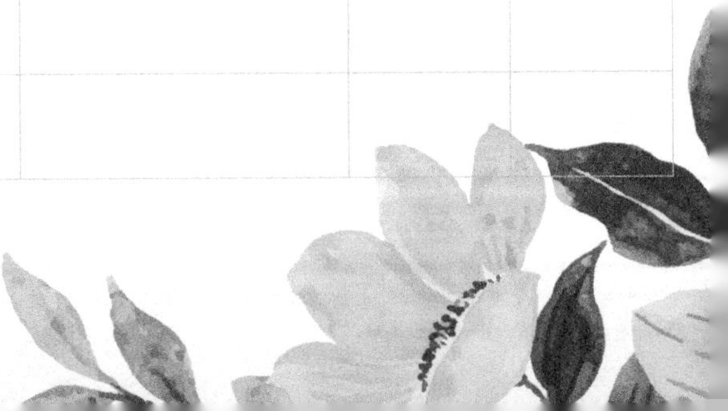

Medication Log

Month & Year ______________________

Week Starting ______________________

Reminders ______________________

Notes ______________________

Medication							
Dosage							
Day	Time						
Mon	AM						
	Mid						
	PM						
Tue	AM						
	Mid						
	PM						
Wed	AM						
	Mid						
	PM						
Thu	AM						
	Mid						
	PM						
Fri	AM						
	Mid						
	PM						
Sat	AM						
	Mid						
	PM						
Sun	AM						
	Mid						
	PM						

Medication Log

Month & Year ______________________

Week Starting ______________________

Reminders ______________________

Notes ______________________

Medication							
Dosage							
Day	**Time**						
Mon	AM						
	Mid						
	PM						
Tue	AM						
	Mid						
	PM						
Wed	AM						
	Mid						
	PM						
Thu	AM						
	Mid						
	PM						
Fri	AM						
	Mid						
	PM						
Sat	AM						
	Mid						
	PM						
Sun	AM						
	Mid						
	PM						

Medication Log

Month & Year ______________________

Week Starting ______________________

Reminders ______________________

Notes ______________________

Medication							
Dosage							
Day	**Time**						
Mon	AM						
	Mid						
	PM						
Tue	AM						
	Mid						
	PM						
Wed	AM						
	Mid						
	PM						
Thu	AM						
	Mid						
	PM						
Fri	AM						
	Mid						
	PM						
Sat	AM						
	Mid						
	PM						
Sun	AM						
	Mid						
	PM						

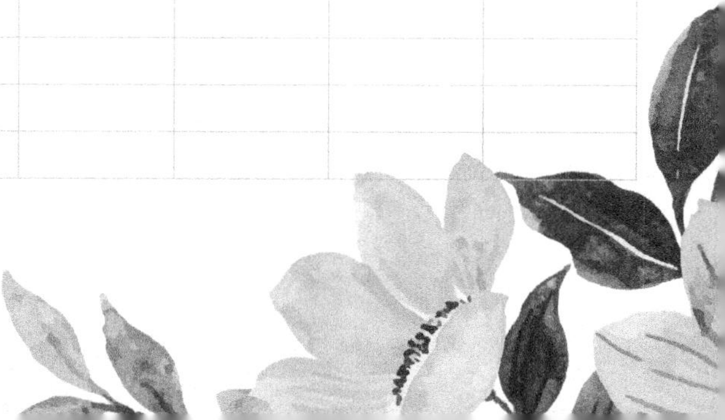

Medication Log

Month & Year ______________________________

Week Starting ______________________________

Reminders ______________________________

Notes ______________________________

Medication							
Dosage							
Day	**Time**						
Mon	AM						
	Mid						
	PM						
Tue	AM						
	Mid						
	PM						
Wed	AM						
	Mid						
	PM						
Thu	AM						
	Mid						
	PM						
Fri	AM						
	Mid						
	PM						
Sat	AM						
	Mid						
	PM						
Sun	AM						
	Mid						
	PM						

Medication Log

Month & Year ______________________________

Week Starting ______________________________

Reminders ______________________________

Notes ______________________________

Medication							
Dosage							
Day	Time						
Mon	AM						
	Mid						
	PM						
Tue	AM						
	Mid						
	PM						
Wed	AM						
	Mid						
	PM						
Thu	AM						
	Mid						
	PM						
Fri	AM						
	Mid						
	PM						
Sat	AM						
	Mid						
	PM						
Sun	AM						
	Mid						
	PM						

Medication Log

Month & Year ______________________________

Week Starting ______________________________

Reminders ______________________________

Notes ______________________________

Medication							
Dosage							
Day	Time						
Mon	AM						
	Mid						
	PM						
Tue	AM						
	Mid						
	PM						
Wed	AM						
	Mid						
	PM						
Thu	AM						
	Mid						
	PM						
Fri	AM						
	Mid						
	PM						
Sat	AM						
	Mid						
	PM						
Sun	AM						
	Mid						
	PM						

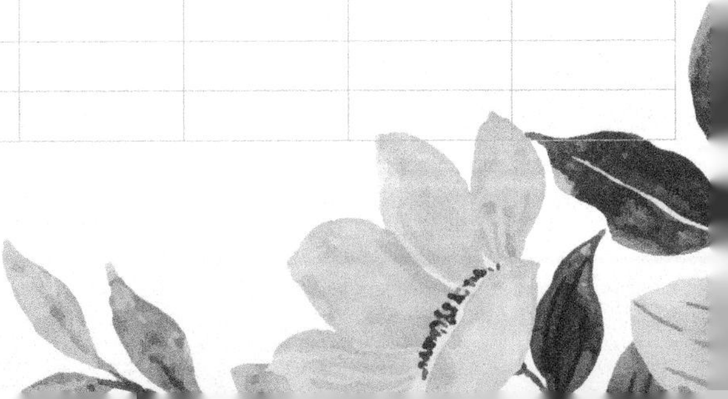

Medication Log

Month & Year ______________________________

Week Starting ______________________________

Reminders ______________________________

Notes ______________________________

Medication							
Dosage							
Day	**Time**						
Mon	AM						
	Mid						
	PM						
Tue	AM						
	Mid						
	PM						
Wed	AM						
	Mid						
	PM						
Thu	AM						
	Mid						
	PM						
Fri	AM						
	Mid						
	PM						
Sat	AM						
	Mid						
	PM						
Sun	AM						
	Mid						
	PM						

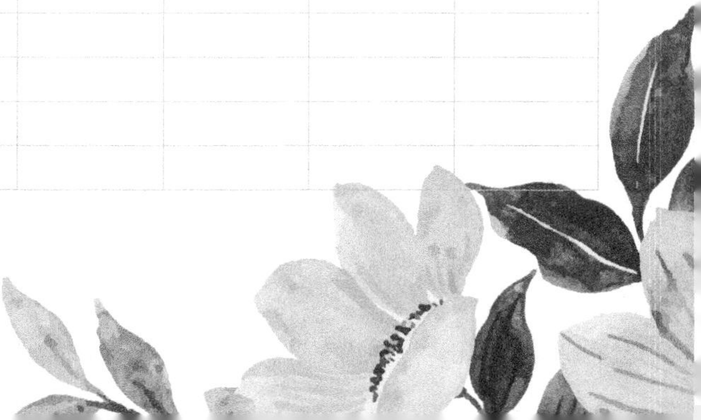

Medication Log

Month & Year ______________________________

Week Starting ______________________________

Reminders ______________________________

Notes ______________________________

Medication							
Dosage							
Day	**Time**						
Mon	AM						
	Mid						
	PM						
Tue	AM						
	Mid						
	PM						
Wed	AM						
	Mid						
	PM						
Thu	AM						
	Mid						
	PM						
Fri	AM						
	Mid						
	PM						
Sat	AM						
	Mid						
	PM						
Sun	AM						
	Mid						
	PM						

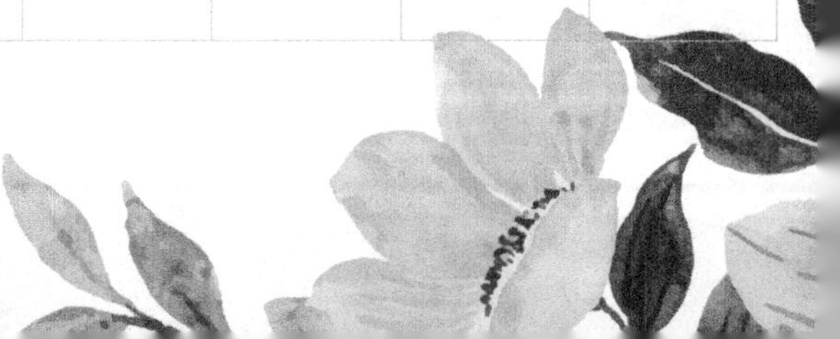

Medication Log

Month & Year ______________________

Week Starting ______________________

Reminders ______________________

Notes ______________________

Medication							
Dosage							
Day	**Time**						
Mon	AM						
	Mid						
	PM						
Tue	AM						
	Mid						
	PM						
Wed	AM						
	Mid						
	PM						
Thu	AM						
	Mid						
	PM						
Fri	AM						
	Mid						
	PM						
Sat	AM						
	Mid						
	PM						
Sun	AM						
	Mid						
	PM						

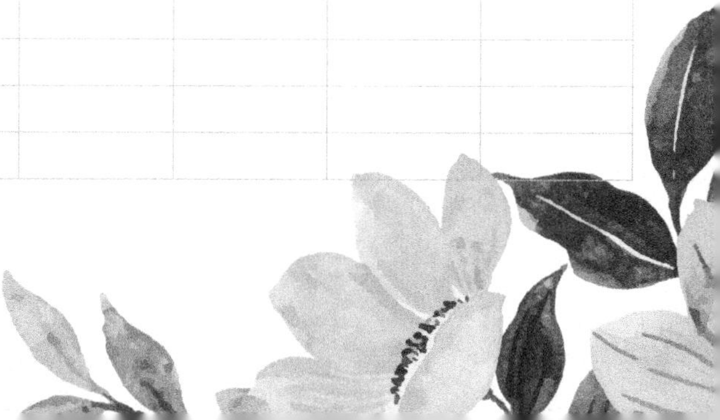

Medication Log

Month & Year ______________________________

Week Starting ______________________________

Reminders ______________________________

Notes ______________________________

Medication							
Dosage							
Day	**Time**						
Mon	AM						
	Mid						
	PM						
Tue	AM						
	Mid						
	PM						
Wed	AM						
	Mid						
	PM						
Thu	AM						
	Mid						
	PM						
Fri	AM						
	Mid						
	PM						
Sat	AM						
	Mid						
	PM						
Sun	AM						
	Mid						
	PM						

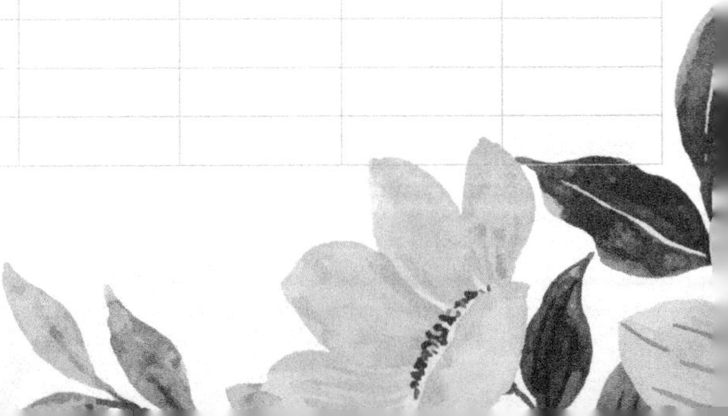

Medication Log

Month & Year ______________________

Week Starting ______________________

Reminders ______________________

Notes ______________________

Medication							
Dosage							
Day	**Time**						
Mon	AM						
	Mid						
	PM						
Tue	AM						
	Mid						
	PM						
Wed	AM						
	Mid						
	PM						
Thu	AM						
	Mid						
	PM						
Fri	AM						
	Mid						
	PM						
Sat	AM						
	Mid						
	PM						
Sun	AM						
	Mid						
	PM						

Medication Log

Month & Year ______________________________

Week Starting ______________________________

Reminders ______________________________

Notes ______________________________

Medication							
Dosage							
Day	**Time**						
Mon	AM						
	Mid						
	PM						
Tue	AM						
	Mid						
	PM						
Wed	AM						
	Mid						
	PM						
Thu	AM						
	Mid						
	PM						
Fri	AM						
	Mid						
	PM						
Sat	AM						
	Mid						
	PM						
Sun	AM						
	Mid						
	PM						

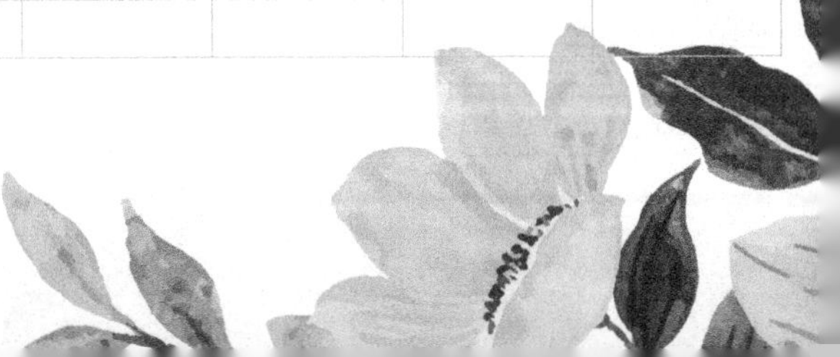

Medication Log

Month & Year ____________________

Week Starting ____________________

Reminders ____________________

Notes ____________________

Medication							
Dosage							
Day	**Time**						
Mon	AM						
	Mid						
	PM						
Tue	AM						
	Mid						
	PM						
Wed	AM						
	Mid						
	PM						
Thu	AM						
	Mid						
	PM						
Fri	AM						
	Mid						
	PM						
Sat	AM						
	Mid						
	PM						
Sun	AM						
	Mid						
	PM						

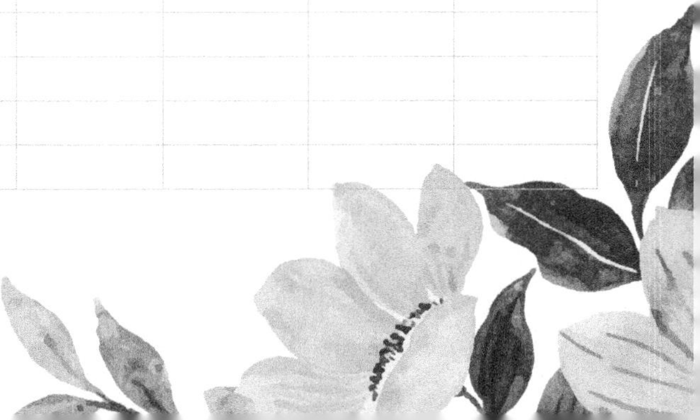

Medication Log

Month & Year ____________________

Week Starting ____________________

Reminders ____________________

Notes ____________________

Medication							
Dosage							
Day	**Time**						
Mon	AM						
	Mid						
	PM						
Tue	AM						
	Mid						
	PM						
Wed	AM						
	Mid						
	PM						
Thu	AM						
	Mid						
	PM						
Fri	AM						
	Mid						
	PM						
Sat	AM						
	Mid						
	PM						
Sun	AM						
	Mid						
	PM						

Medication Log

Month & Year ____________________

Week Starting ____________________

Reminders ____________________

Notes ____________________

Medication							
Dosage							
Day	**Time**						
Mon	AM						
	Mid						
	PM						
Tue	AM						
	Mid						
	PM						
Wed	AM						
	Mid						
	PM						
Thu	AM						
	Mid						
	PM						
Fri	AM						
	Mid						
	PM						
Sat	AM						
	Mid						
	PM						
Sun	AM						
	Mid						
	PM						

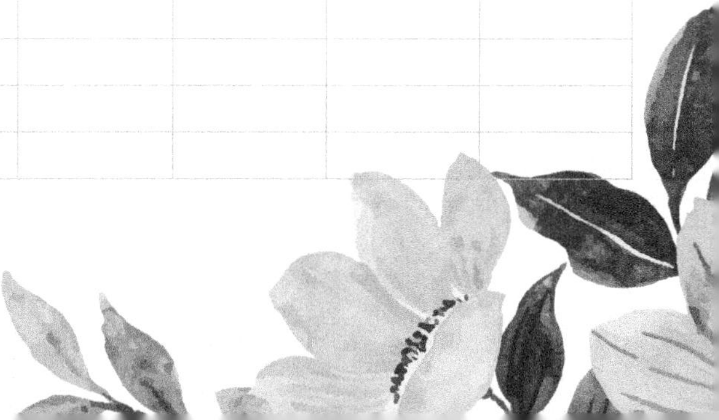

Medication Log

Month & Year ______________________________

Week Starting ______________________________

Reminders ______________________________

Notes ______________________________

Medication							
Dosage							
Day	Time						
Mon	AM						
	Mid						
	PM						
Tue	AM						
	Mid						
	PM						
Wed	AM						
	Mid						
	PM						
Thu	AM						
	Mid						
	PM						
Fri	AM						
	Mid						
	PM						
Sat	AM						
	Mid						
	PM						
Sun	AM						
	Mid						
	PM						

Medication Log

Month & Year ______________________

Week Starting ______________________

Reminders ______________________

Notes ______________________

Medication							
Dosage							
Day	**Time**						
Mon	AM						
	Mid						
	PM						
Tue	AM						
	Mid						
	PM						
Wed	AM						
	Mid						
	PM						
Thu	AM						
	Mid						
	PM						
Fri	AM						
	Mid						
	PM						
Sat	AM						
	Mid						
	PM						
Sun	AM						
	Mid						
	PM						

Medication Log

Month & Year ______________________________

Week Starting ______________________________

Reminders ______________________________

Notes ______________________________

Medication							
Dosage							
Day	**Time**						
Mon	AM						
	Mid						
	PM						
Tue	AM						
	Mid						
	PM						
Wed	AM						
	Mid						
	PM						
Thu	AM						
	Mid						
	PM						
Fri	AM						
	Mid						
	PM						
Sat	AM						
	Mid						
	PM						
Sun	AM						
	Mid						
	PM						

Medication Log

Month & Year ______________________________

Week Starting ______________________________

Reminders ______________________________

Notes ______________________________

Medication							
Dosage							
Day	**Time**						
Mon	AM						
	Mid						
	PM						
Tue	AM						
	Mid						
	PM						
Wed	AM						
	Mid						
	PM						
Thu	AM						
	Mid						
	PM						
Fri	AM						
	Mid						
	PM						
Sat	AM						
	Mid						
	PM						
Sun	AM						
	Mid						
	PM						

Medication Log

Month & Year ______________________

Week Starting ______________________

Reminders ______________________

Notes ______________________

Medication							
Dosage							
Day	Time						
Mon	AM						
	Mid						
	PM						
Tue	AM						
	Mid						
	PM						
Wed	AM						
	Mid						
	PM						
Thu	AM						
	Mid						
	PM						
Fri	AM						
	Mid						
	PM						
Sat	AM						
	Mid						
	PM						
Sun	AM						
	Mid						
	PM						

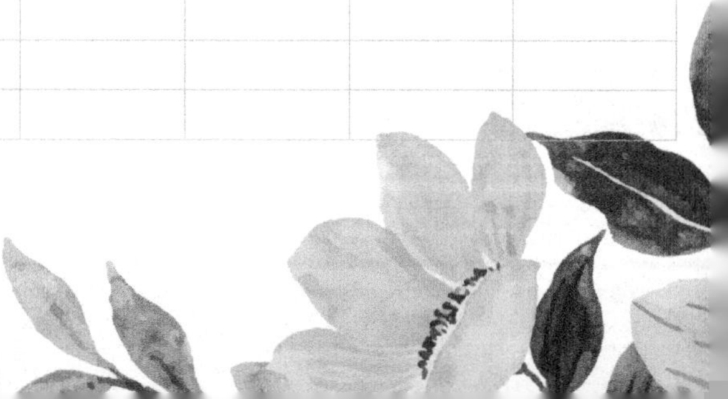

Medication Log

Month & Year ______________________________

Week Starting ______________________________

Reminders ______________________________

Notes ______________________________

Medication							
Dosage							
Day	**Time**						
Mon	AM						
	Mid						
	PM						
Tue	AM						
	Mid						
	PM						
Wed	AM						
	Mid						
	PM						
Thu	AM						
	Mid						
	PM						
Fri	AM						
	Mid						
	PM						
Sat	AM						
	Mid						
	PM						
Sun	AM						
	Mid						
	PM						

Medication Log

Month & Year ____________________

Week Starting ____________________

Reminders ____________________

Notes ____________________

Medication							
Dosage							
Day	Time						
Mon	AM						
	Mid						
	PM						
Tue	AM						
	Mid						
	PM						
Wed	AM						
	Mid						
	PM						
Thu	AM						
	Mid						
	PM						
Fri	AM						
	Mid						
	PM						
Sat	AM						
	Mid						
	PM						
Sun	AM						
	Mid						
	PM						

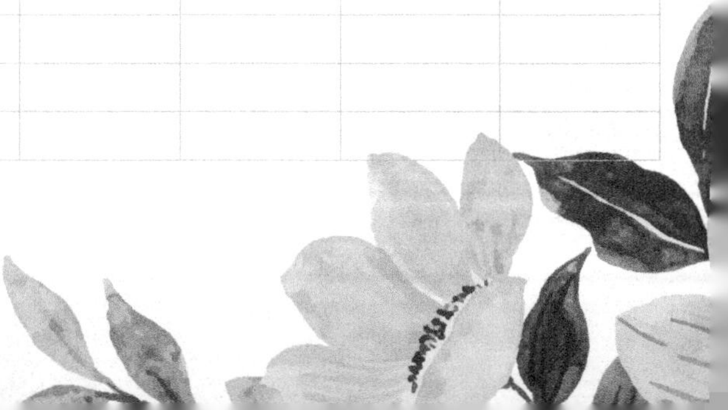

Medication Log

Month & Year ______________________

Week Starting ______________________

Reminders ______________________

Notes ______________________

Medication							
Dosage							
Day	**Time**						
Mon	AM						
	Mid						
	PM						
Tue	AM						
	Mid						
	PM						
Wed	AM						
	Mid						
	PM						
Thu	AM						
	Mid						
	PM						
Fri	AM						
	Mid						
	PM						
Sat	AM						
	Mid						
	PM						
Sun	AM						
	Mid						
	PM						

Medication Log

Month & Year ______________________

Week Starting ______________________

Reminders ______________________

Notes ______________________

Medication							
Dosage							
Day	**Time**						
Mon	AM						
	Mid						
	PM						
Tue	AM						
	Mid						
	PM						
Wed	AM						
	Mid						
	PM						
Thu	AM						
	Mid						
	PM						
Fri	AM						
	Mid						
	PM						
Sat	AM						
	Mid						
	PM						
Sun	AM						
	Mid						
	PM						

Medication Log

Month & Year ______________________________

Week Starting ______________________________

Reminders ______________________________

Notes ______________________________

Medication							
Dosage							
Day	**Time**						
Mon	AM						
	Mid						
	PM						
Tue	AM						
	Mid						
	PM						
Wed	AM						
	Mid						
	PM						
Thu	AM						
	Mid						
	PM						
Fri	AM						
	Mid						
	PM						
Sat	AM						
	Mid						
	PM						
Sun	AM						
	Mid						
	PM						

Medication Log

Month & Year ______________________________

Week Starting ______________________________

Reminders ______________________________

Notes ______________________________

Medication							
Dosage							
Day	Time						
Mon	AM						
	Mid						
	PM						
Tue	AM						
	Mid						
	PM						
Wed	AM						
	Mid						
	PM						
Thu	AM						
	Mid						
	PM						
Fri	AM						
	Mid						
	PM						
Sat	AM						
	Mid						
	PM						
Sun	AM						
	Mid						
	PM						

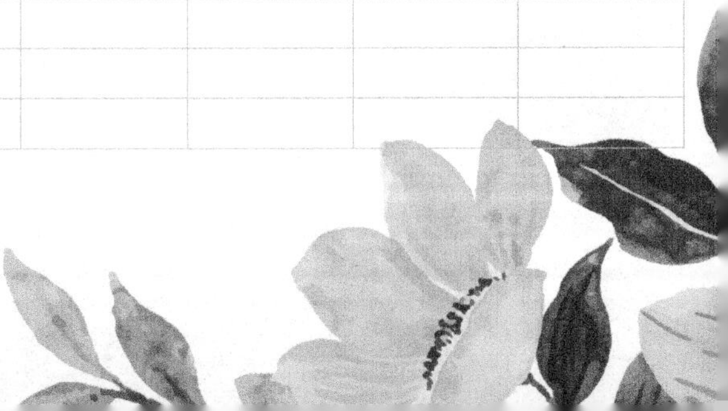

Medication Log

Month & Year ________________________

Week Starting ________________________

Reminders ________________________

Notes ________________________

Medication							
Dosage							
Day	**Time**						
Mon	AM						
	Mid						
	PM						
Tue	AM						
	Mid						
	PM						
Wed	AM						
	Mid						
	PM						
Thu	AM						
	Mid						
	PM						
Fri	AM						
	Mid						
	PM						
Sat	AM						
	Mid						
	PM						
Sun	AM						
	Mid						
	PM						

Medication Log

Month & Year ______________________

Week Starting ______________________

Reminders ______________________

Notes ______________________

Medication							
Dosage							
Day	**Time**						
Mon	AM						
	Mid						
	PM						
Tue	AM						
	Mid						
	PM						
Wed	AM						
	Mid						
	PM						
Thu	AM						
	Mid						
	PM						
Fri	AM						
	Mid						
	PM						
Sat	AM						
	Mid						
	PM						
Sun	AM						
	Mid						
	PM						

Medication Log

Month & Year ______________________

Week Starting ______________________

Reminders ______________________

Notes ______________________

Medication							
Dosage							
Day	**Time**						
Mon	AM						
	Mid						
	PM						
Tue	AM						
	Mid						
	PM						
Wed	AM						
	Mid						
	PM						
Thu	AM						
	Mid						
	PM						
Fri	AM						
	Mid						
	PM						
Sat	AM						
	Mid						
	PM						
Sun	AM						
	Mid						
	PM						

Medication Log

Month & Year ______________________________

Week Starting ______________________________

Reminders ______________________________

Notes ______________________________

Medication							
Dosage							
Day	**Time**						
Mon	AM						
	Mid						
	PM						
Tue	AM						
	Mid						
	PM						
Wed	AM						
	Mid						
	PM						
Thu	AM						
	Mid						
	PM						
Fri	AM						
	Mid						
	PM						
Sat	AM						
	Mid						
	PM						
Sun	AM						
	Mid						
	PM						

Medication Log

Month & Year	______________________
Week Starting	______________________
Reminders	______________________
Notes	______________________

Medication							
Dosage							
Day	**Time**						
Mon	AM						
	Mid						
	PM						
Tue	AM						
	Mid						
	PM						
Wed	AM						
	Mid						
	PM						
Thu	AM						
	Mid						
	PM						
Fri	AM						
	Mid						
	PM						
Sat	AM						
	Mid						
	PM						
Sun	AM						
	Mid						
	PM						

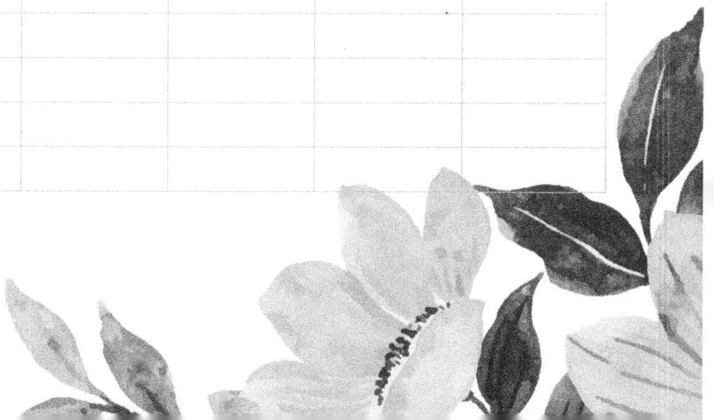

Medication Log

Month & Year ______________________________

Week Starting ______________________________

Reminders ______________________________

Notes ______________________________

Medication							
Dosage							
Day	**Time**						
Mon	AM						
	Mid						
	PM						
Tue	AM						
	Mid						
	PM						
Wed	AM						
	Mid						
	PM						
Thu	AM						
	Mid						
	PM						
Fri	AM						
	Mid						
	PM						
Sat	AM						
	Mid						
	PM						
Sun	AM						
	Mid						
	PM						

Medication Log

Month & Year ______________________________

Week Starting ______________________________

Reminders ______________________________

Notes ______________________________

Medication							
Dosage							
Day	**Time**						
Mon	AM						
	Mid						
	PM						
Tue	AM						
	Mid						
	PM						
Wed	AM						
	Mid						
	PM						
Thu	AM						
	Mid						
	PM						
Fri	AM						
	Mid						
	PM						
Sat	AM						
	Mid						
	PM						
Sun	AM						
	Mid						
	PM						

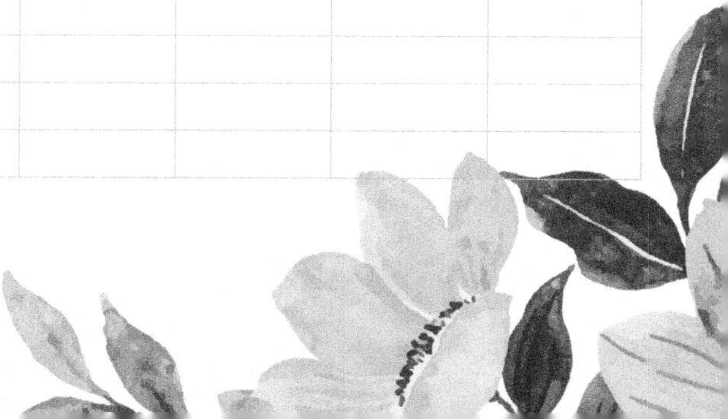

Medication Log

Month & Year ____________________

Week Starting ____________________

Reminders ____________________

Notes ____________________

Medication							
Dosage							
Day	**Time**						
Mon	AM						
	Mid						
	PM						
Tue	AM						
	Mid						
	PM						
Wed	AM						
	Mid						
	PM						
Thu	AM						
	Mid						
	PM						
Fri	AM						
	Mid						
	PM						
Sat	AM						
	Mid						
	PM						
Sun	AM						
	Mid						
	PM						

Medication Log

Month & Year ______________________

Week Starting ______________________

Reminders ______________________

Notes ______________________

Medication							
Dosage							
Day	**Time**						
Mon	AM						
	Mid						
	PM						
Tue	AM						
	Mid						
	PM						
Wed	AM						
	Mid						
	PM						
Thu	AM						
	Mid						
	PM						
Fri	AM						
	Mid						
	PM						
Sat	AM						
	Mid						
	PM						
Sun	AM						
	Mid						
	PM						

Medication Log

Month & Year ______________________________

Week Starting ______________________________

Reminders ______________________________

Notes ______________________________

Medication							
Dosage							
Day	Time						
Mon	AM						
	Mid						
	PM						
Tue	AM						
	Mid						
	PM						
Wed	AM						
	Mid						
	PM						
Thu	AM						
	Mid						
	PM						
Fri	AM						
	Mid						
	PM						
Sat	AM						
	Mid						
	PM						
Sun	AM						
	Mid						
	PM						

Medication Log

Month & Year ______________________________

Week Starting ______________________________

Reminders ______________________________

Notes ______________________________

Medication							
Dosage							
Day	Time						
Mon	AM						
	Mid						
	PM						
Tue	AM						
	Mid						
	PM						
Wed	AM						
	Mid						
	PM						
Thu	AM						
	Mid						
	PM						
Fri	AM						
	Mid						
	PM						
Sat	AM						
	Mid						
	PM						
Sun	AM						
	Mid						
	PM						

Medication Log

Month & Year ______________________

Week Starting ______________________

Reminders ______________________

Notes ______________________

Medication							
Dosage							
Day	Time						
Mon	AM						
	Mid						
	PM						
Tue	AM						
	Mid						
	PM						
Wed	AM						
	Mid						
	PM						
Thu	AM						
	Mid						
	PM						
Fri	AM						
	Mid						
	PM						
Sat	AM						
	Mid						
	PM						
Sun	AM						
	Mid						
	PM						

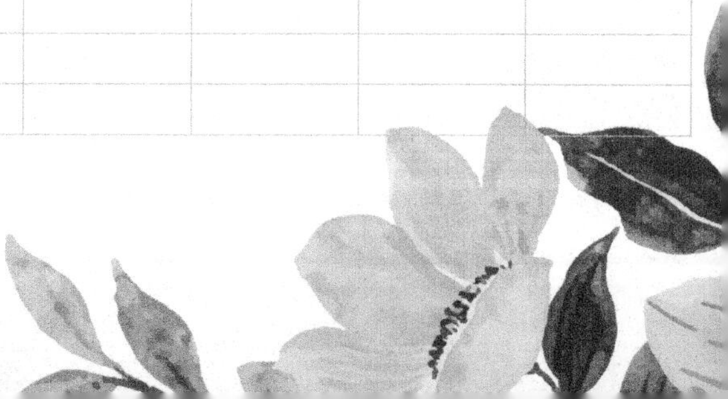

Medication Log

Month & Year ______________________

Week Starting ______________________

Reminders ______________________

Notes ______________________

Medication							
Dosage							
Day	**Time**						
Mon	AM						
	Mid						
	PM						
Tue	AM						
	Mid						
	PM						
Wed	AM						
	Mid						
	PM						
Thu	AM						
	Mid						
	PM						
Fri	AM						
	Mid						
	PM						
Sat	AM						
	Mid						
	PM						
Sun	AM						
	Mid						
	PM						

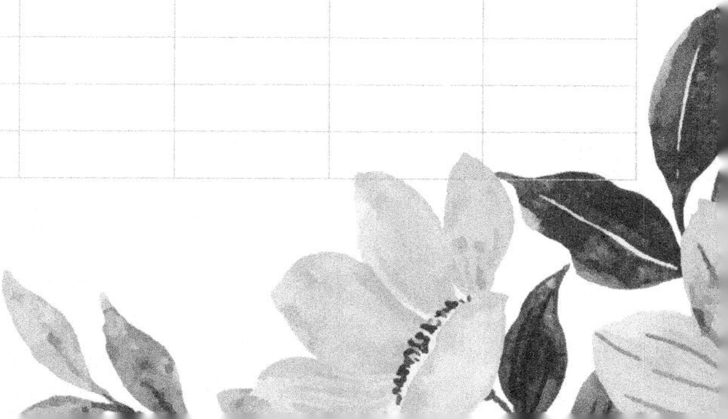

Medication Log

Month & Year ______________________

Week Starting ______________________

Reminders ______________________

Notes ______________________

Medication							
Dosage							
Day	**Time**						
Mon	AM						
	Mid						
	PM						
Tue	AM						
	Mid						
	PM						
Wed	AM						
	Mid						
	PM						
Thu	AM						
	Mid						
	PM						
Fri	AM						
	Mid						
	PM						
Sat	AM						
	Mid						
	PM						
Sun	AM						
	Mid						
	PM						

Medication Log

Month & Year ______________________________

Week Starting ______________________________

Reminders ______________________________

Notes ______________________________

Medication							
Dosage							
Day	**Time**						
Mon	AM						
	Mid						
	PM						
Tue	AM						
	Mid						
	PM						
Wed	AM						
	Mid						
	PM						
Thu	AM						
	Mid						
	PM						
Fri	AM						
	Mid						
	PM						
Sat	AM						
	Mid						
	PM						
Sun	AM						
	Mid						
	PM						

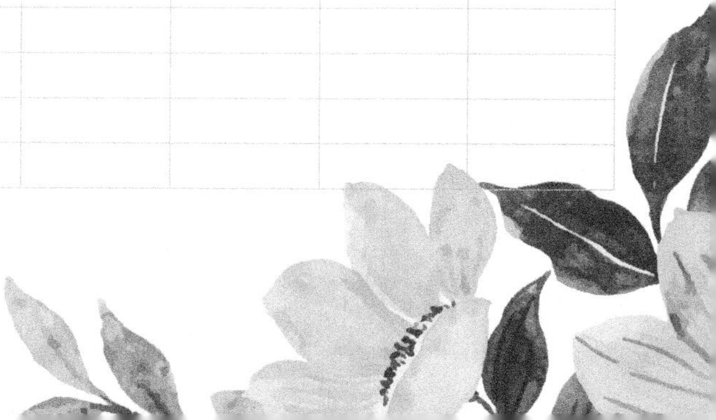

Medication Log

Month & Year ______________________________

Week Starting ______________________________

Reminders ______________________________

Notes ______________________________

Medication							
Dosage							
Day	**Time**						
Mon	AM						
	Mid						
	PM						
Tue	AM						
	Mid						
	PM						
Wed	AM						
	Mid						
	PM						
Thu	AM						
	Mid						
	PM						
Fri	AM						
	Mid						
	PM						
Sat	AM						
	Mid						
	PM						
Sun	AM						
	Mid						
	PM						

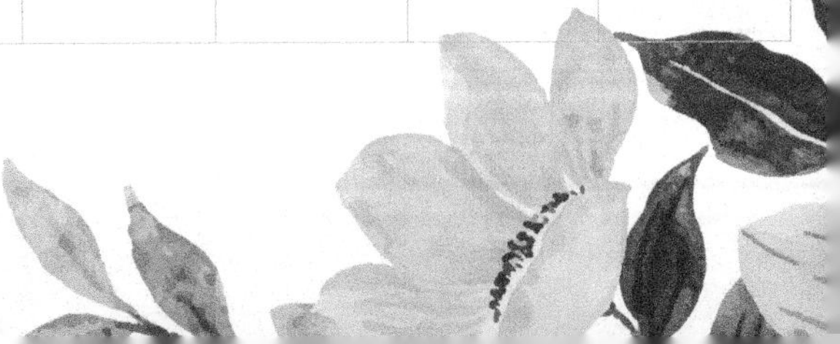

Medication Log

Month & Year ______________________________

Week Starting ______________________________

Reminders ______________________________

Notes ______________________________

Medication							
Dosage							
Day	Time						
Mon	AM						
	Mid						
	PM						
Tue	AM						
	Mid						
	PM						
Wed	AM						
	Mid						
	PM						
Thu	AM						
	Mid						
	PM						
Fri	AM						
	Mid						
	PM						
Sat	AM						
	Mid						
	PM						
Sun	AM						
	Mid						
	PM						

Medication Log

Month & Year ______________________

Week Starting ______________________

Reminders ______________________

Notes ______________________

Medication							
Dosage							
Day	Time						
Mon	AM						
	Mid						
	PM						
Tue	AM						
	Mid						
	PM						
Wed	AM						
	Mid						
	PM						
Thu	AM						
	Mid						
	PM						
Fri	AM						
	Mid						
	PM						
Sat	AM						
	Mid						
	PM						
Sun	AM						
	Mid						
	PM						

Medication Log

Month & Year ____________________

Week Starting ____________________

Reminders ____________________

Notes ____________________

Medication							
Dosage							
Day	**Time**						
Mon	AM						
	Mid						
	PM						
Tue	AM						
	Mid						
	PM						
Wed	AM						
	Mid						
	PM						
Thu	AM						
	Mid						
	PM						
Fri	AM						
	Mid						
	PM						
Sat	AM						
	Mid						
	PM						
Sun	AM						
	Mid						
	PM						

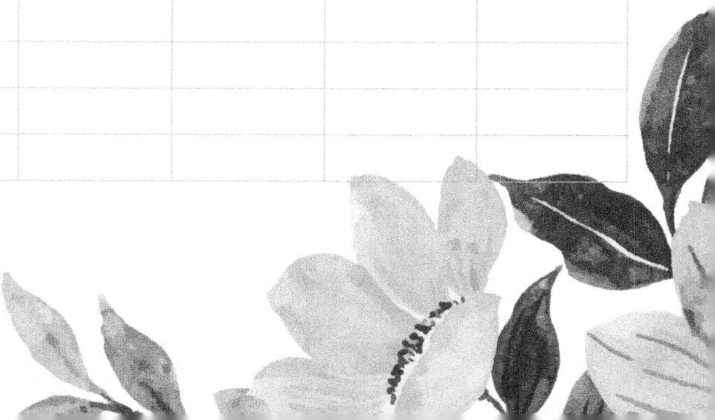

Medication Log

Month & Year ______________________________

Week Starting ______________________________

Reminders ______________________________

Notes ______________________________

Medication							
Dosage							
Day	**Time**						
Mon	AM						
	Mid						
	PM						
Tue	AM						
	Mid						
	PM						
Wed	AM						
	Mid						
	PM						
Thu	AM						
	Mid						
	PM						
Fri	AM						
	Mid						
	PM						
Sat	AM						
	Mid						
	PM						
Sun	AM						
	Mid						
	PM						

Medication Log

Month & Year ____________________

Week Starting ____________________

Reminders ____________________

Notes ____________________

Medication							
Dosage							
Day	Time						
Mon	AM						
	Mid						
	PM						
Tue	AM						
	Mid						
	PM						
Wed	AM						
	Mid						
	PM						
Thu	AM						
	Mid						
	PM						
Fri	AM						
	Mid						
	PM						
Sat	AM						
	Mid						
	PM						
Sun	AM						
	Mid						
	PM						

Medication Log

Month & Year ______________________

Week Starting ______________________

Reminders ______________________

Notes ______________________

Medication							
Dosage							
Day	**Time**						
Mon	AM						
	Mid						
	PM						
Tue	AM						
	Mid						
	PM						
Wed	AM						
	Mid						
	PM						
Thu	AM						
	Mid						
	PM						
Fri	AM						
	Mid						
	PM						
Sat	AM						
	Mid						
	PM						
Sun	AM						
	Mid						
	PM						

Medication Log

Month & Year ____________________

Week Starting ____________________

Reminders ____________________

Notes ____________________

Medication							
Dosage							
Day	**Time**						
Mon	AM						
	Mid						
	PM						
Tue	AM						
	Mid						
	PM						
Wed	AM						
	Mid						
	PM						
Thu	AM						
	Mid						
	PM						
Fri	AM						
	Mid						
	PM						
Sat	AM						
	Mid						
	PM						
Sun	AM						
	Mid						
	PM						

Medication Log

Month & Year ____________________

Week Starting ____________________

Reminders ____________________

Notes ____________________

Medication							
Dosage							
Day	**Time**						
Mon	AM						
	Mid						
	PM						
Tue	AM						
	Mid						
	PM						
Wed	AM						
	Mid						
	PM						
Thu	AM						
	Mid						
	PM						
Fri	AM						
	Mid						
	PM						
Sat	AM						
	Mid						
	PM						
Sun	AM						
	Mid						
	PM						

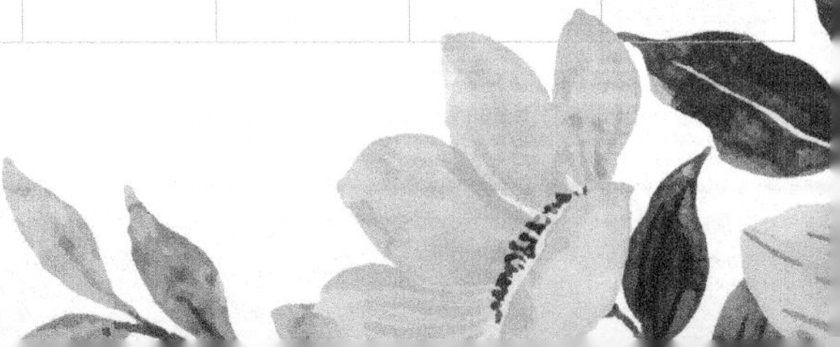

Medication Log

Month & Year ______________________

Week Starting ______________________

Reminders ______________________

Notes ______________________

Medication							
Dosage							
Day	Time						
Mon	AM						
	Mid						
	PM						
Tue	AM						
	Mid						
	PM						
Wed	AM						
	Mid						
	PM						
Thu	AM						
	Mid						
	PM						
Fri	AM						
	Mid						
	PM						
Sat	AM						
	Mid						
	PM						
Sun	AM						
	Mid						
	PM						

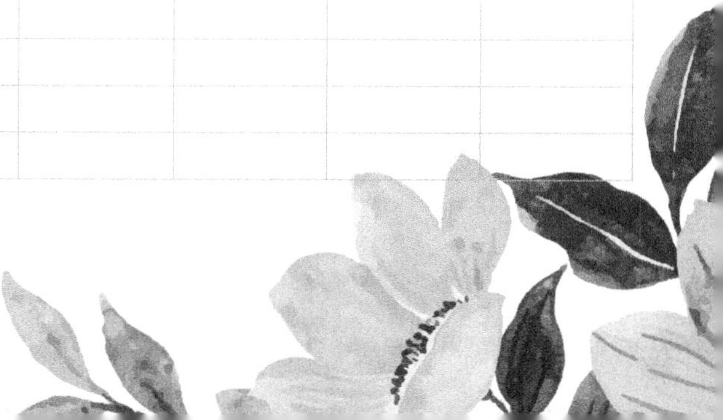

Medication Log

Month & Year ______________________

Week Starting ______________________

Reminders ______________________

Notes ______________________

Medication							
Dosage							
Day	Time						
Mon	AM						
	Mid						
	PM						
Tue	AM						
	Mid						
	PM						
Wed	AM						
	Mid						
	PM						
Thu	AM						
	Mid						
	PM						
Fri	AM						
	Mid						
	PM						
Sat	AM						
	Mid						
	PM						
Sun	AM						
	Mid						
	PM						

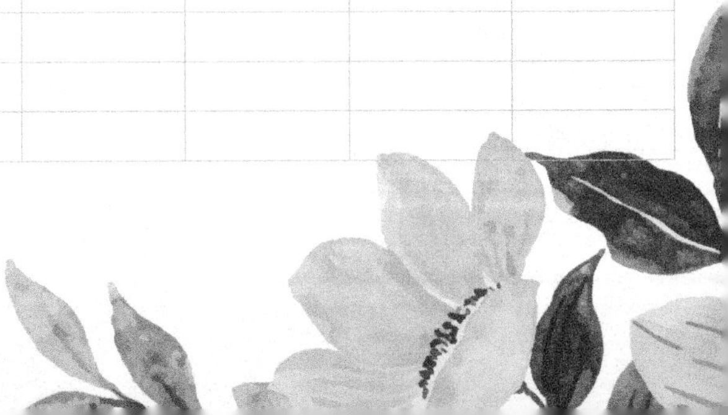

Medication Log

Month & Year ______________________________

Week Starting ______________________________

Reminders ______________________________

Notes ______________________________

Medication							
Dosage							
Day	Time						
Mon	AM						
	Mid						
	PM						
Tue	AM						
	Mid						
	PM						
Wed	AM						
	Mid						
	PM						
Thu	AM						
	Mid						
	PM						
Fri	AM						
	Mid						
	PM						
Sat	AM						
	Mid						
	PM						
Sun	AM						
	Mid						
	PM						

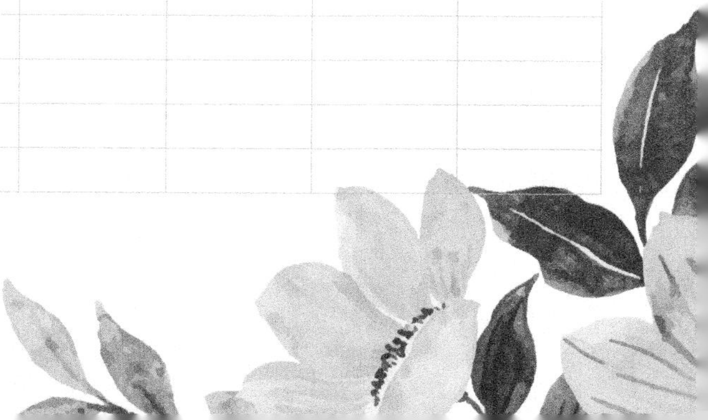

Medication Log

Month & Year ____________________

Week Starting ____________________

Reminders ____________________

Notes ____________________

Medication							
Dosage							
Day	**Time**						
Mon	AM						
	Mid						
	PM						
Tue	AM						
	Mid						
	PM						
Wed	AM						
	Mid						
	PM						
Thu	AM						
	Mid						
	PM						
Fri	AM						
	Mid						
	PM						
Sat	AM						
	Mid						
	PM						
Sun	AM						
	Mid						
	PM						

Medication Log

Month & Year ______________________

Week Starting ______________________

Reminders ______________________

Notes ______________________

Medication							
Dosage							
Day	Time						
Mon	AM						
	Mid						
	PM						
Tue	AM						
	Mid						
	PM						
Wed	AM						
	Mid						
	PM						
Thu	AM						
	Mid						
	PM						
Fri	AM						
	Mid						
	PM						
Sat	AM						
	Mid						
	PM						
Sun	AM						
	Mid						
	PM						

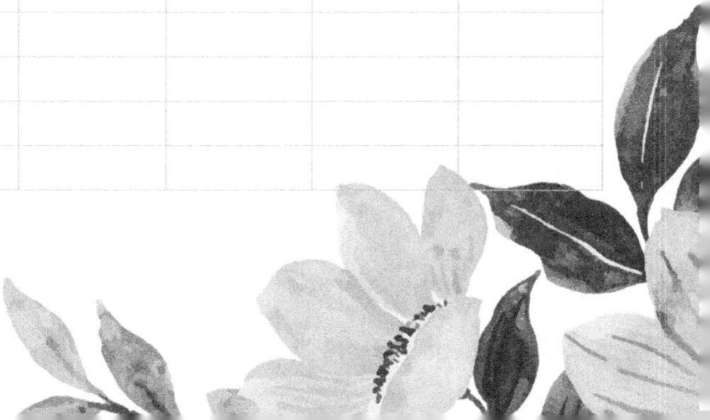

Medication Log

Month & Year ______________________________

Week Starting ______________________________

Reminders ______________________________

Notes ______________________________

Medication							
Dosage							
Day	Time						
Mon	AM						
	Mid						
	PM						
Tue	AM						
	Mid						
	PM						
Wed	AM						
	Mid						
	PM						
Thu	AM						
	Mid						
	PM						
Fri	AM						
	Mid						
	PM						
Sat	AM						
	Mid						
	PM						
Sun	AM						
	Mid						
	PM						

Medication Log

Month & Year ______________________________

Week Starting ______________________________

Reminders ______________________________

Notes ______________________________

Medication							
Dosage							
Day	Time						
Mon	AM						
	Mid						
	PM						
Tue	AM						
	Mid						
	PM						
Wed	AM						
	Mid						
	PM						
Thu	AM						
	Mid						
	PM						
Fri	AM						
	Mid						
	PM						
Sat	AM						
	Mid						
	PM						
Sun	AM						
	Mid						
	PM						

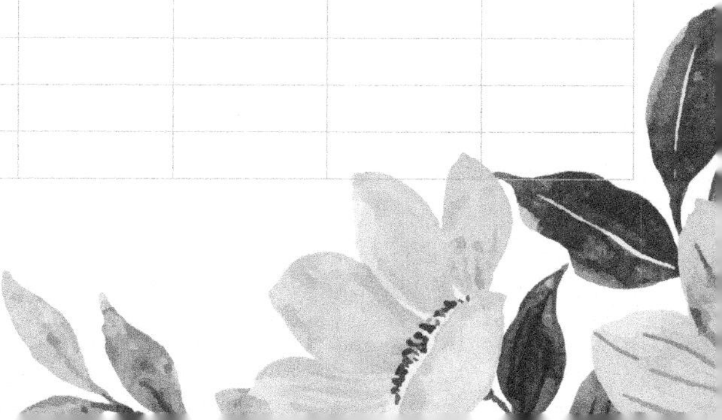

Medication Log

Month & Year ______________________________

Week Starting ______________________________

Reminders ______________________________

Notes ______________________________

Medication							
Dosage							
Day	**Time**						
Mon	AM						
	Mid						
	PM						
Tue	AM						
	Mid						
	PM						
Wed	AM						
	Mid						
	PM						
Thu	AM						
	Mid						
	PM						
Fri	AM						
	Mid						
	PM						
Sat	AM						
	Mid						
	PM						
Sun	AM						
	Mid						
	PM						

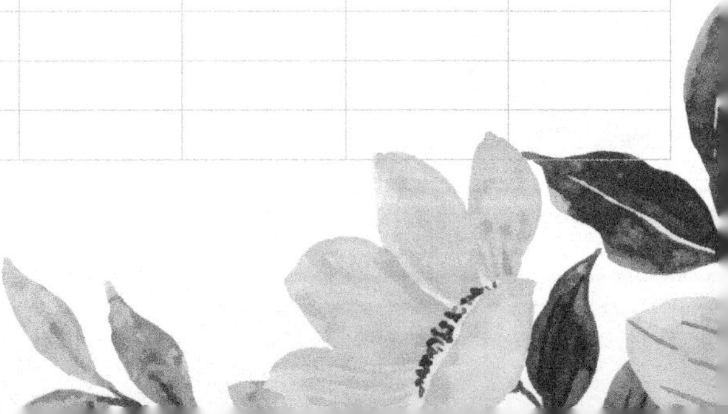

Medication Log

Month & Year ______________________

Week Starting ______________________

Reminders ______________________

Notes ______________________

Medication							
Dosage							
Day	**Time**						
Mon	AM						
	Mid						
	PM						
Tue	AM						
	Mid						
	PM						
Wed	AM						
	Mid						
	PM						
Thu	AM						
	Mid						
	PM						
Fri	AM						
	Mid						
	PM						
Sat	AM						
	Mid						
	PM						
Sun	AM						
	Mid						
	PM						

Medication Log

Month & Year ______________________________

Week Starting ______________________________

Reminders ______________________________

Notes ______________________________

Medication							
Dosage							
Day	Time						
Mon	AM						
	Mid						
	PM						
Tue	AM						
	Mid						
	PM						
Wed	AM						
	Mid						
	PM						
Thu	AM						
	Mid						
	PM						
Fri	AM						
	Mid						
	PM						
Sat	AM						
	Mid						
	PM						
Sun	AM						
	Mid						
	PM						

Medication Log

Month & Year ______________________

Week Starting ______________________

Reminders ______________________

Notes ______________________

Medication							
Dosage							
Day	**Time**						
Mon	AM						
	Mid						
	PM						
Tue	AM						
	Mid						
	PM						
Wed	AM						
	Mid						
	PM						
Thu	AM						
	Mid						
	PM						
Fri	AM						
	Mid						
	PM						
Sat	AM						
	Mid						
	PM						
Sun	AM						
	Mid						
	PM						

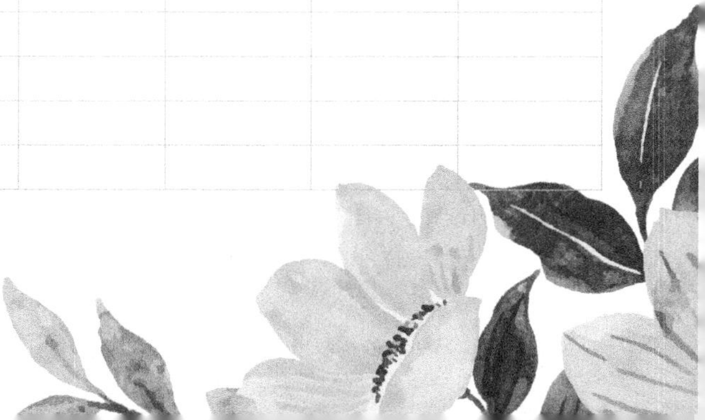

Medication Log

Month & Year ______________________________

Week Starting ______________________________

Reminders ______________________________

Notes ______________________________

Medication							
Dosage							
Day	Time						
Mon	AM						
	Mid						
	PM						
Tue	AM						
	Mid						
	PM						
Wed	AM						
	Mid						
	PM						
Thu	AM						
	Mid						
	PM						
Fri	AM						
	Mid						
	PM						
Sat	AM						
	Mid						
	PM						
Sun	AM						
	Mid						
	PM						

Medication Log

Month & Year ____________________

Week Starting ____________________

Reminders ____________________

Notes ____________________

Medication							
Dosage							
Day	**Time**						
Mon	AM						
	Mid						
	PM						
Tue	AM						
	Mid						
	PM						
Wed	AM						
	Mid						
	PM						
Thu	AM						
	Mid						
	PM						
Fri	AM						
	Mid						
	PM						
Sat	AM						
	Mid						
	PM						
Sun	AM						
	Mid						
	PM						

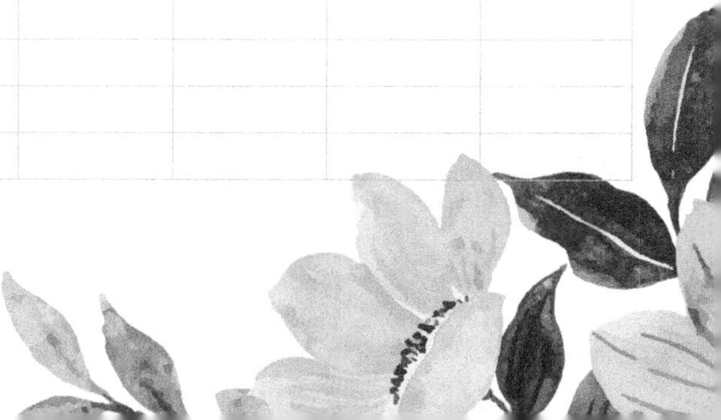

Medication Log

Month & Year ____________________

Week Starting ____________________

Reminders ____________________

Notes ____________________

Medication							
Dosage							
Day	**Time**						
Mon	AM						
	Mid						
	PM						
Tue	AM						
	Mid						
	PM						
Wed	AM						
	Mid						
	PM						
Thu	AM						
	Mid						
	PM						
Fri	AM						
	Mid						
	PM						
Sat	AM						
	Mid						
	PM						
Sun	AM						
	Mid						
	PM						

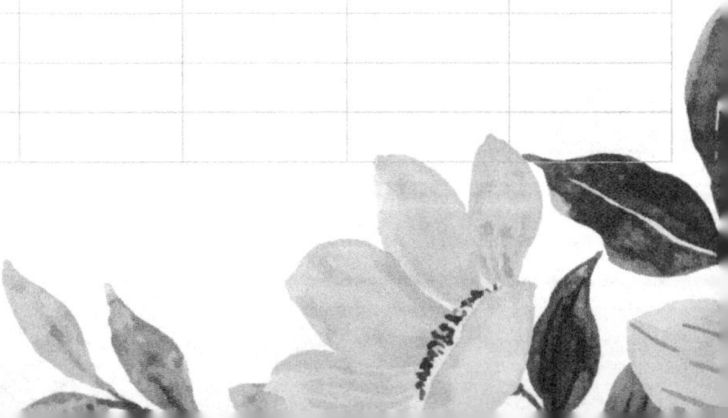

Medication Log

Month & Year ______________________________

Week Starting ______________________________

Reminders ______________________________

Notes ______________________________

Medication							
Dosage							
Day	**Time**						
Mon	AM						
	Mid						
	PM						
Tue	AM						
	Mid						
	PM						
Wed	AM						
	Mid						
	PM						
Thu	AM						
	Mid						
	PM						
Fri	AM						
	Mid						
	PM						
Sat	AM						
	Mid						
	PM						
Sun	AM						
	Mid						
	PM						

Medication Log

Month & Year ______________________

Week Starting ______________________

Reminders ______________________

Notes ______________________

Medication							
Dosage							
Day	**Time**						
Mon	AM						
	Mid						
	PM						
Tue	AM						
	Mid						
	PM						
Wed	AM						
	Mid						
	PM						
Thu	AM						
	Mid						
	PM						
Fri	AM						
	Mid						
	PM						
Sat	AM						
	Mid						
	PM						
Sun	AM						
	Mid						
	PM						

Medication Log

Month & Year ______________________

Week Starting ______________________

Reminders ______________________

Notes ______________________

Medication							
Dosage							
Day	Time						
Mon	AM						
	Mid						
	PM						
Tue	AM						
	Mid						
	PM						
Wed	AM						
	Mid						
	PM						
Thu	AM						
	Mid						
	PM						
Fri	AM						
	Mid						
	PM						
Sat	AM						
	Mid						
	PM						
Sun	AM						
	Mid						
	PM						

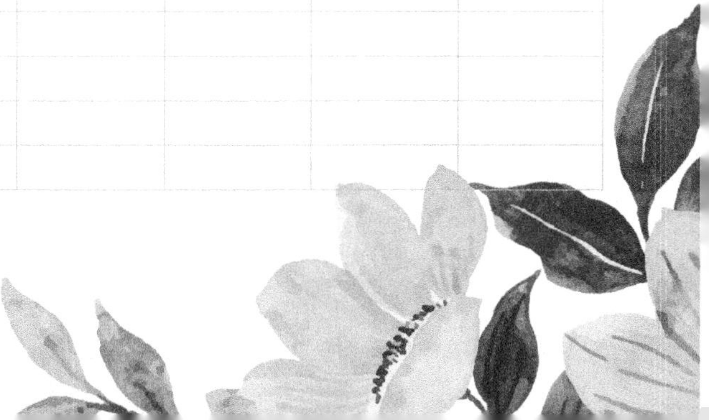

Medication Log

Month & Year ______________________

Week Starting ______________________

Reminders ______________________

Notes ______________________

Medication							
Dosage							
Day	Time						
Mon	AM						
	Mid						
	PM						
Tue	AM						
	Mid						
	PM						
Wed	AM						
	Mid						
	PM						
Thu	AM						
	Mid						
	PM						
Fri	AM						
	Mid						
	PM						
Sat	AM						
	Mid						
	PM						
Sun	AM						
	Mid						
	PM						

Medication Log

Month & Year ______________________

Week Starting ______________________

Reminders ______________________

Notes ______________________

Medication							
Dosage							
Day	Time						
Mon	AM						
	Mid						
	PM						
Tue	AM						
	Mid						
	PM						
Wed	AM						
	Mid						
	PM						
Thu	AM						
	Mid						
	PM						
Fri	AM						
	Mid						
	PM						
Sat	AM						
	Mid						
	PM						
Sun	AM						
	Mid						
	PM						

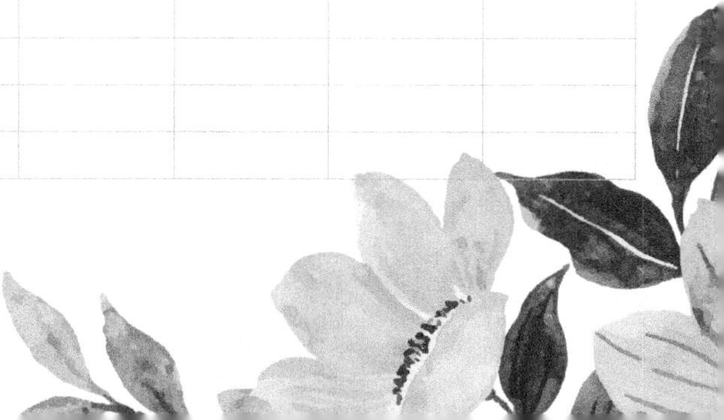

Medication Log

Month & Year ______________________________

Week Starting ______________________________

Reminders ______________________________

Notes ______________________________

Medication							
Dosage							
Day	**Time**						
Mon	AM						
	Mid						
	PM						
Tue	AM						
	Mid						
	PM						
Wed	AM						
	Mid						
	PM						
Thu	AM						
	Mid						
	PM						
Fri	AM						
	Mid						
	PM						
Sat	AM						
	Mid						
	PM						
Sun	AM						
	Mid						
	PM						

Medication Log

Month & Year ____________________

Week Starting ____________________

Reminders ____________________

Notes ____________________

Medication							
Dosage							
Day	Time						
Mon	AM						
	Mid						
	PM						
Tue	AM						
	Mid						
	PM						
Wed	AM						
	Mid						
	PM						
Thu	AM						
	Mid						
	PM						
Fri	AM						
	Mid						
	PM						
Sat	AM						
	Mid						
	PM						
Sun	AM						
	Mid						
	PM						

Medication Log

Month & Year ______________________

Week Starting ______________________

Reminders ______________________

Notes ______________________

Medication							
Dosage							
Day	Time						
Mon	AM						
	Mid						
	PM						
Tue	AM						
	Mid						
	PM						
Wed	AM						
	Mid						
	PM						
Thu	AM						
	Mid						
	PM						
Fri	AM						
	Mid						
	PM						
Sat	AM						
	Mid						
	PM						
Sun	AM						
	Mid						
	PM						

Medication Log

Month & Year ______________________________

Week Starting ______________________________

Reminders ______________________________

Notes ______________________________

Medication							
Dosage							
Day	**Time**						
Mon	AM						
	Mid						
	PM						
Tue	AM						
	Mid						
	PM						
Wed	AM						
	Mid						
	PM						
Thu	AM						
	Mid						
	PM						
Fri	AM						
	Mid						
	PM						
Sat	AM						
	Mid						
	PM						
Sun	AM						
	Mid						
	PM						

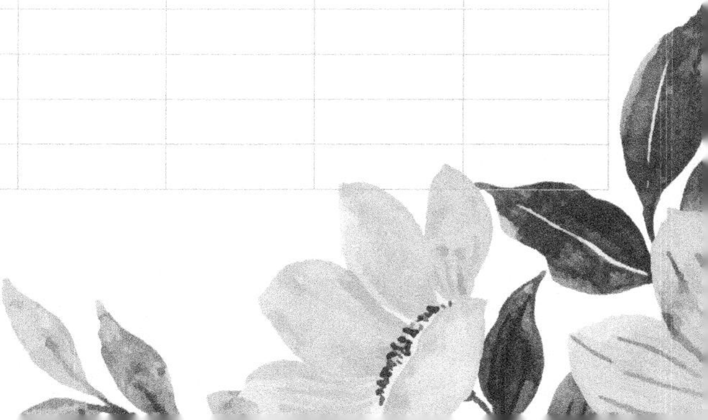

Medication Log

Month & Year ______________________

Week Starting ______________________

Reminders ______________________

Notes ______________________

Medication							
Dosage							
Day	**Time**						
Mon	AM						
	Mid						
	PM						
Tue	AM						
	Mid						
	PM						
Wed	AM						
	Mid						
	PM						
Thu	AM						
	Mid						
	PM						
Fri	AM						
	Mid						
	PM						
Sat	AM						
	Mid						
	PM						
Sun	AM						
	Mid						
	PM						

Made in the USA
Monee, IL
04 November 2026

67379477R00046